Smoking

Aversion Therapy

by E. Nuff & S. Topp

Smoking **Aversion Therapy**

Do you think you are addicted to cigarettes? Sick of thinking about them all the time? Sick of the smell? Had enough of the cost? Are they running your life? Are they ruining your relationships and/or your health? Ready to kick the habit and get your life back? Tried everything to stop?

Finally, here is a way to help you help yourself give up for good. This Smoking Aversion Therapy book is designed to really put you off it. A series of revolting pictures to turn off that old unhealthy habit. Read the instructions carefully, as the method aims to combine several processes to help you free yourself from wanting or needing cigarettes ever again. You have strong willpower. Remember a time when you used it and bring it into play to assist this Aversion Therapy Book.

ISBN-13: 978-1540656094
ISBN-10: 1540656098

IMPORTANT:

read the last 3 pages first.

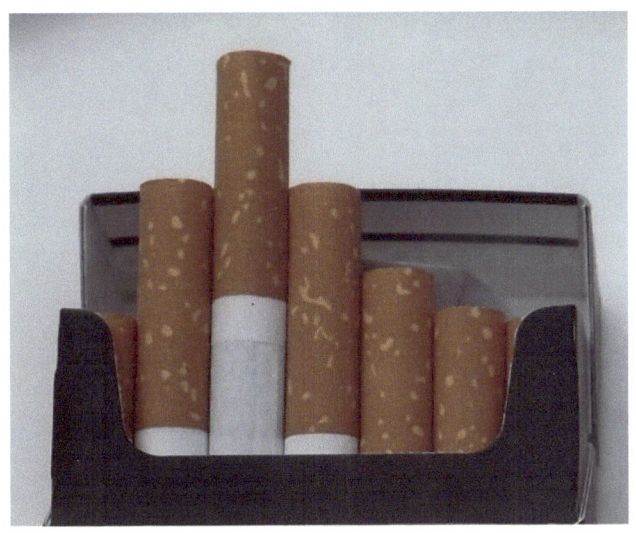

Eeeeek!   Mealy worms!

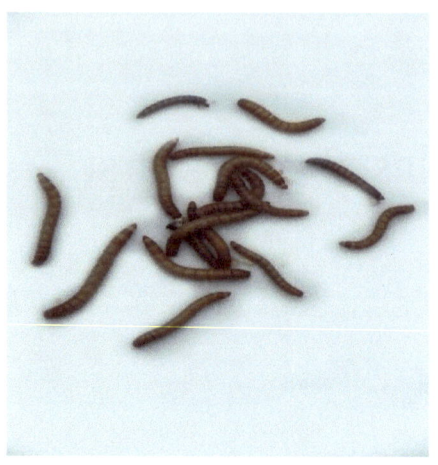

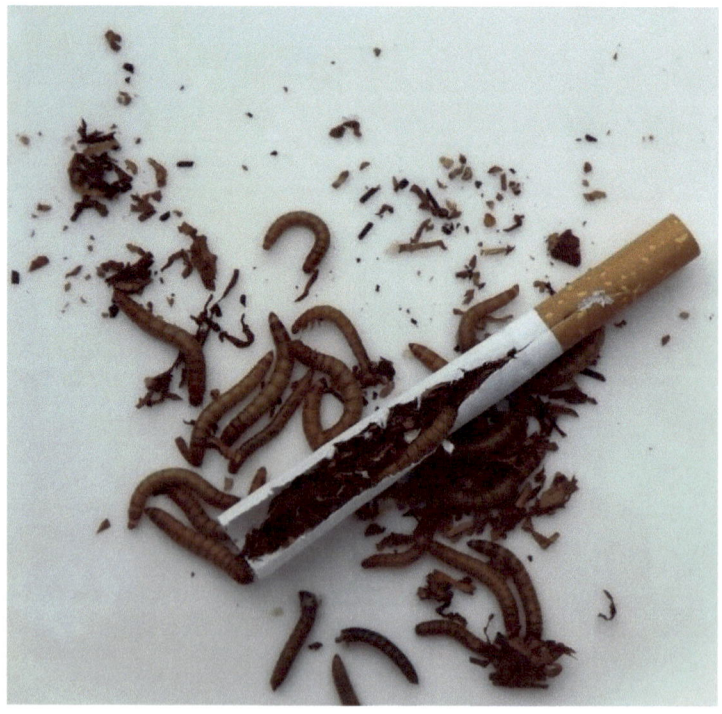

YUCK!　　　cigarettes with mealy worms....

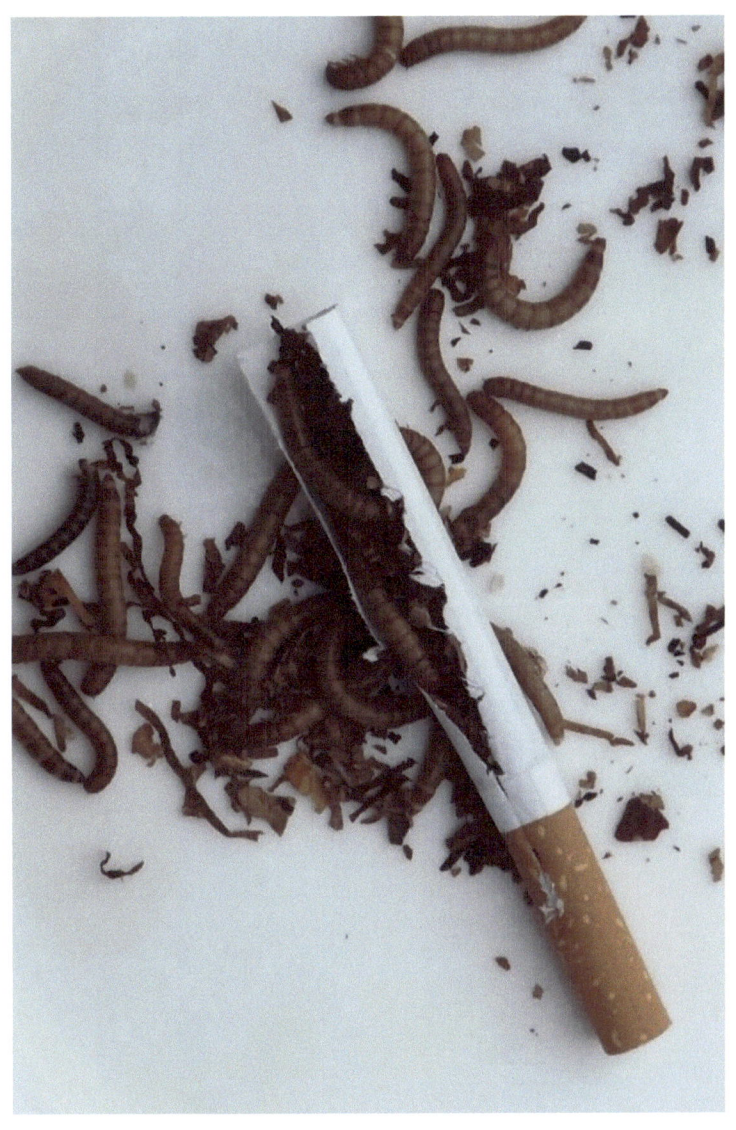

They wriggle. Errrrk!
Tobacco is like floor sweepings. Revolting!

VOMIT!

Remember how it feels, smells and tastes
BEFORE you smoke ....
and just BREATHE air
or drink WATER instead.

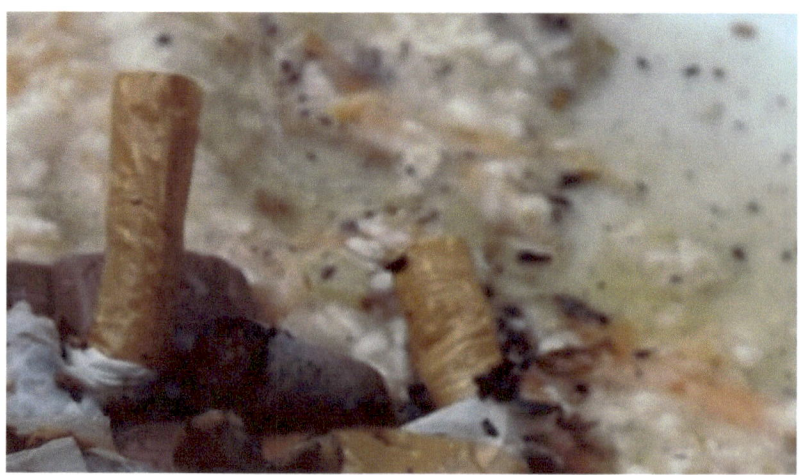

Be reminded of slimy vomit every time you
think about smoking.

Remember the taste and smell. URRGGH!
Remember how sick you felt the first time
you smoked.

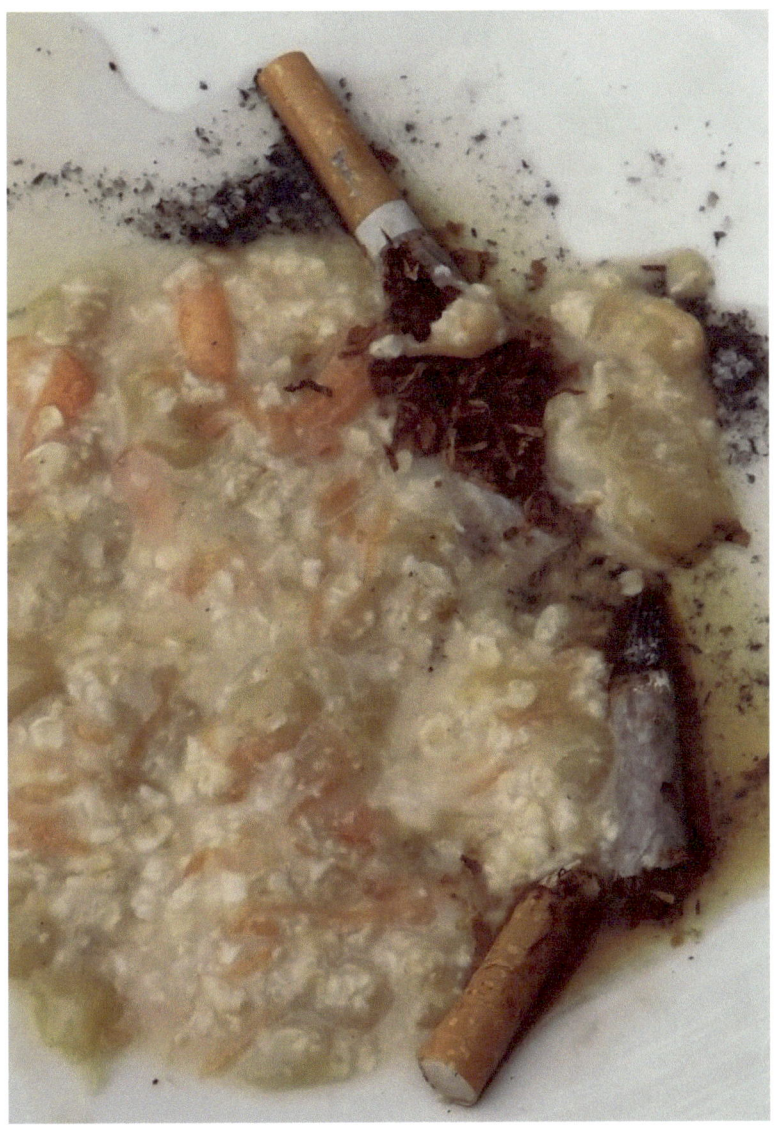

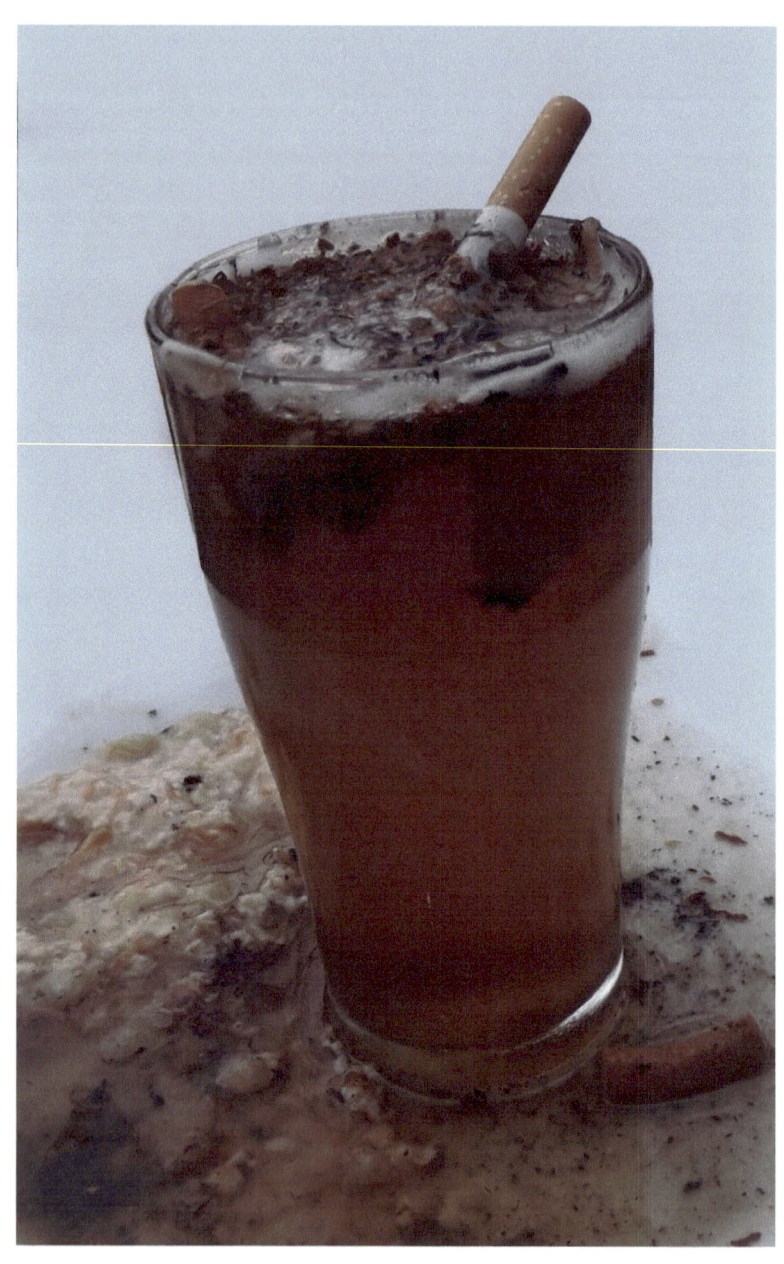

Cigarettes with alcohol: even worse.
Cigarettes RUIN drinks, food, taste...

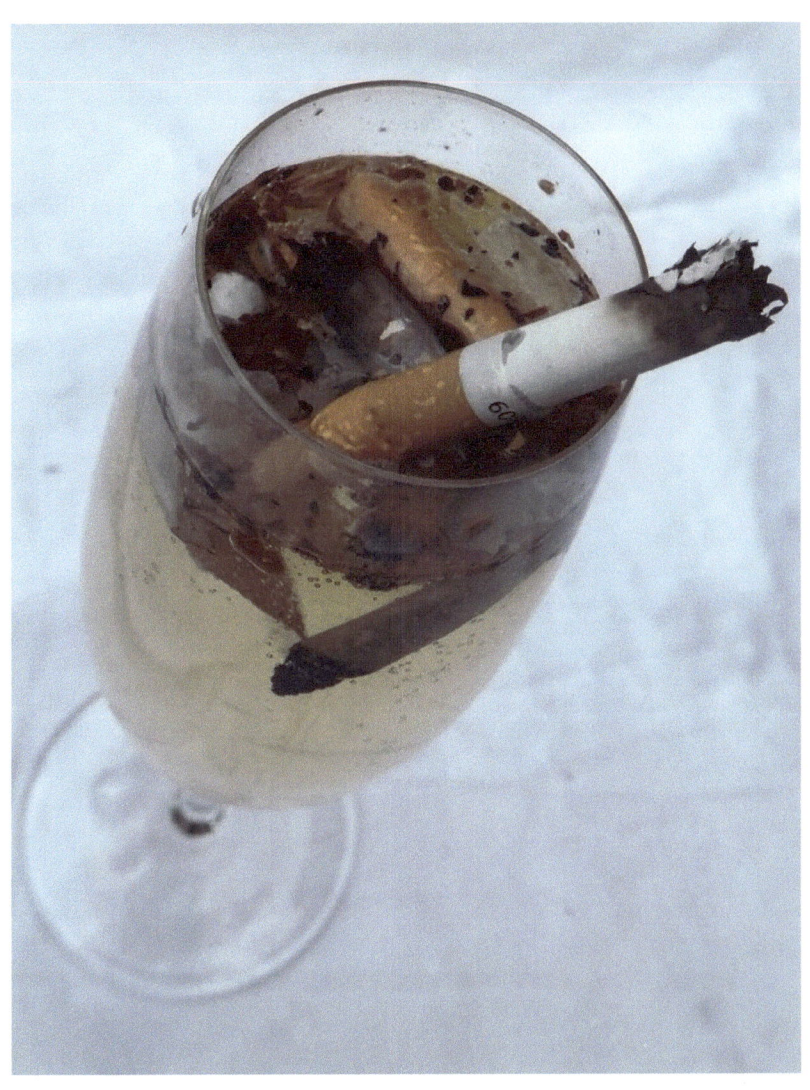

Enjoy life WITHOUT them.

Remember breathing freely?

You can return to health!

Name three things you want
to live for.
Smoking has been a death
sentence for many others.
You deserve better....
and so do your friends and
family.

Passive smoking kills too.

Cigarette filter cut open.

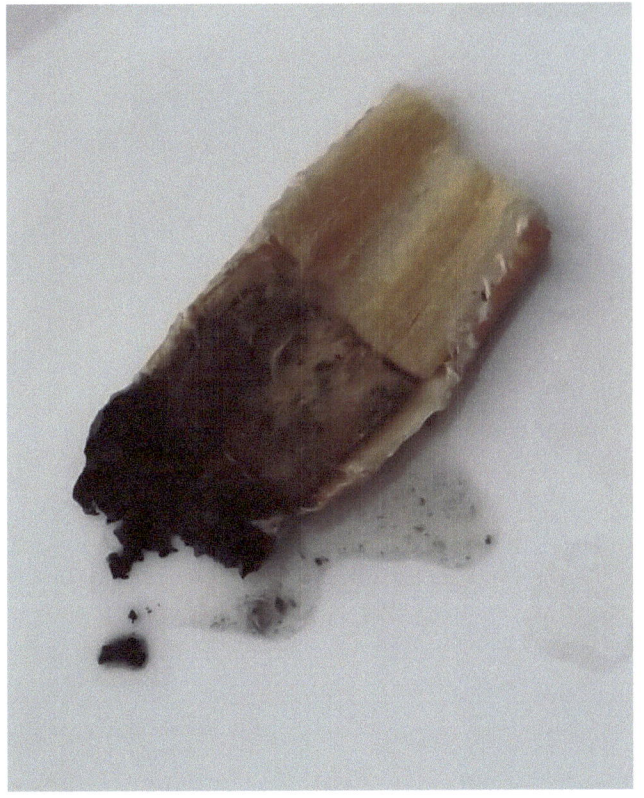

The filter doesn't remove all the tar. A lot of it goes straight into your lungs.

Breathe AIR instead. Whenever you feel stressed, just breathe in relaxation deeply.
Tobacco & tar stain

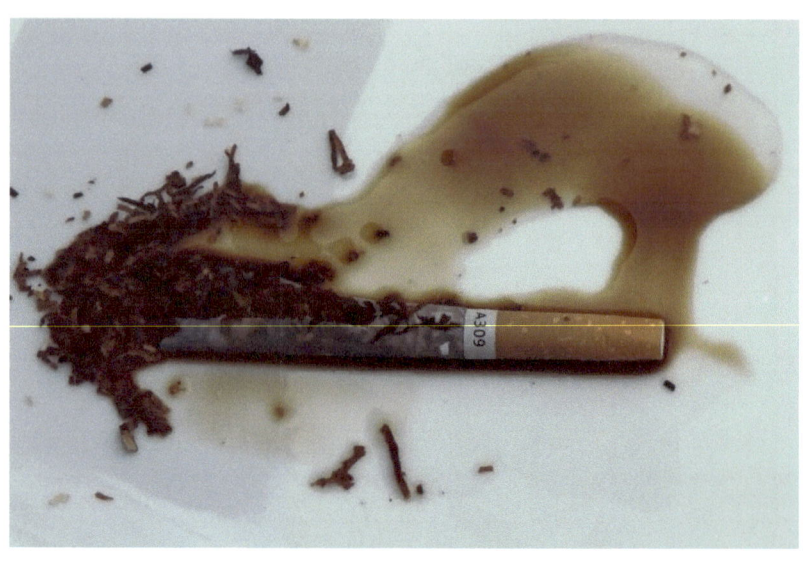

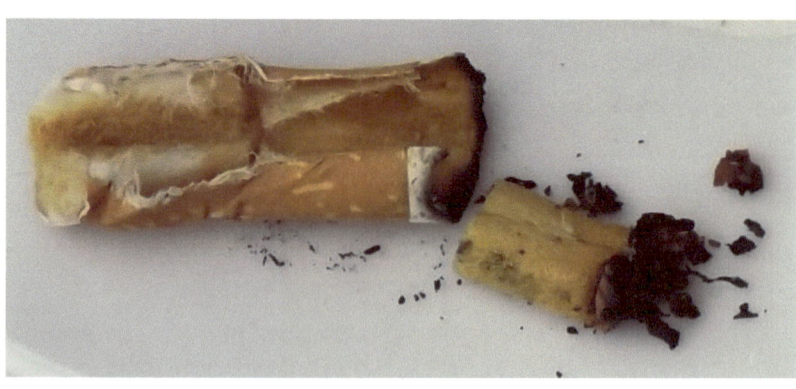

Cigarette Tar can clog lungs. You know it.

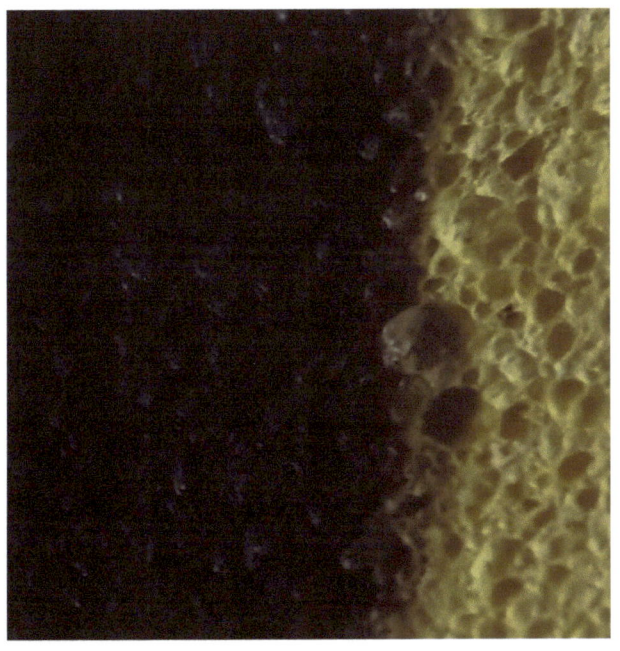

Choose to breathe fresh air instead.
It can relieve stress
better than smoking.

Choose to keep your lungs free of tar.

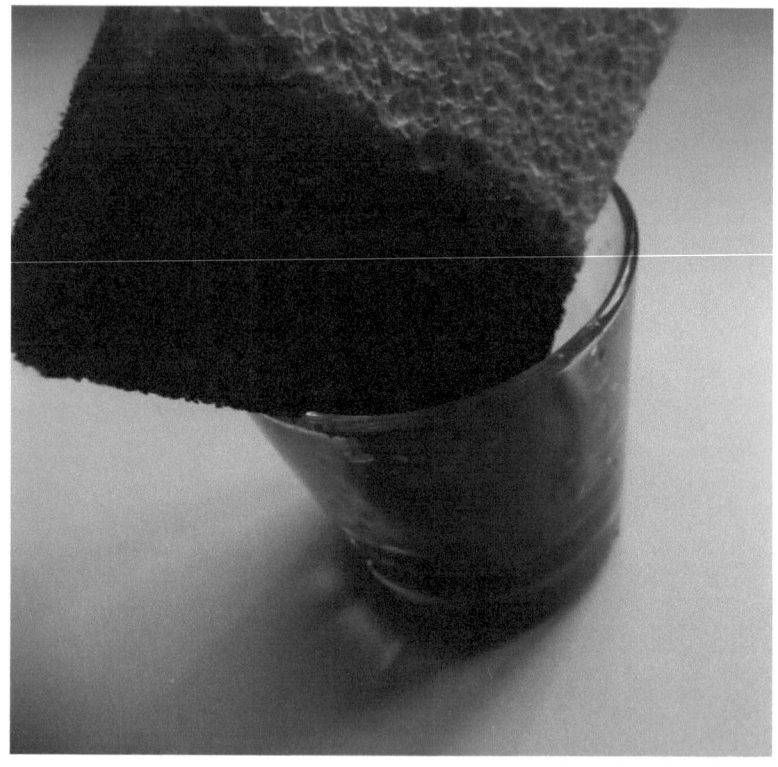

A year after you quit, your lungs will be clearing themselves.

Most of the nicotine will be out of the system within three days. You may feel more energy and find it easier to be calmer without that need nagging at you.

ENOUGH!

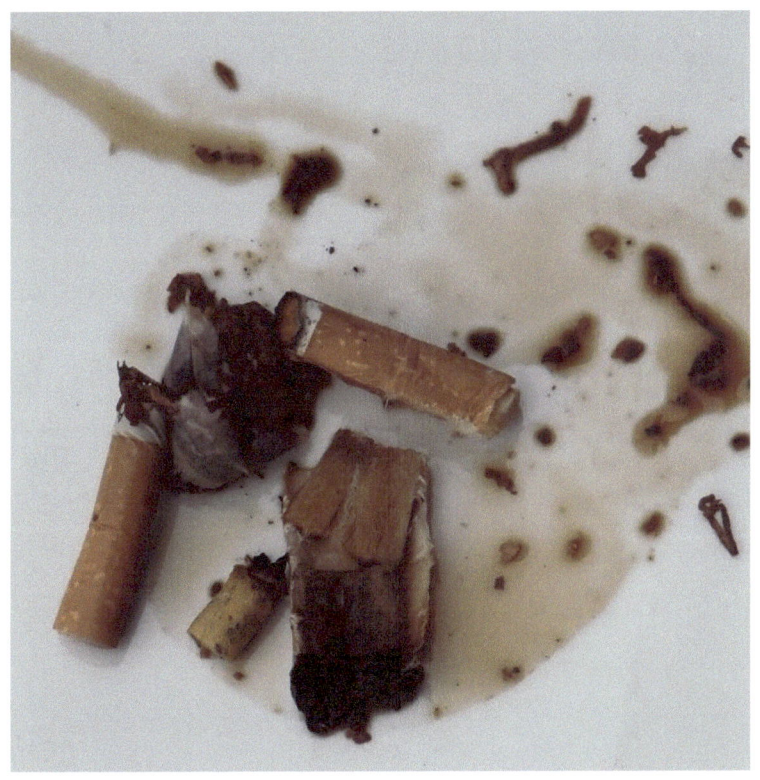

Decide that you have already smoked your last cigarette.

You don't need them any more.

Urrck! You know what that smells like!
Putrid. Old Ash. Damp ashtray.

You are intelligent. Use your intelligence
and stay healthy.

Be glad you have decided not to smoke any
more. You are freeing yourself from that
old habit.   Stop the cycle. Breathe in
deeply: relaxing breaths of air. Exhale
stress. Blow it out as you are used to if you
want.

Drink water.   Imagine it soothing and
relaxing you. It can.

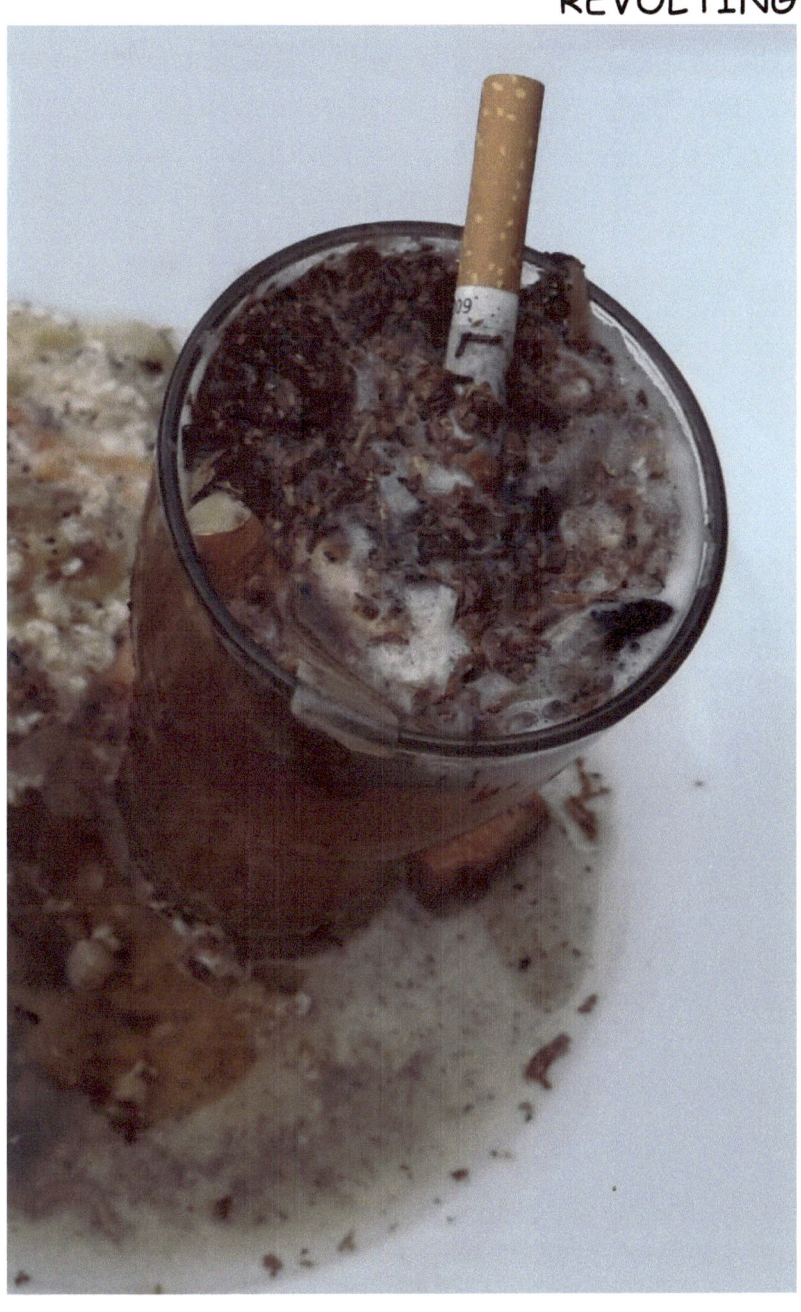

URRGH!
Enough!

You can be free of it. Plan what you will do with the money you save from smoking!

Get a new haircut?
    Your complexion will improve soon.

Take a trip?
    You can save thousands a year now!

Buy some flowers?
    You should soon be able to smell again!

Go out to a restaurant and enjoy the subtle flavours in a salad?
    You should soon regain your taste.

Enjoy your new-found freedom from those old cancer sticks.

URRGH!

Worms !

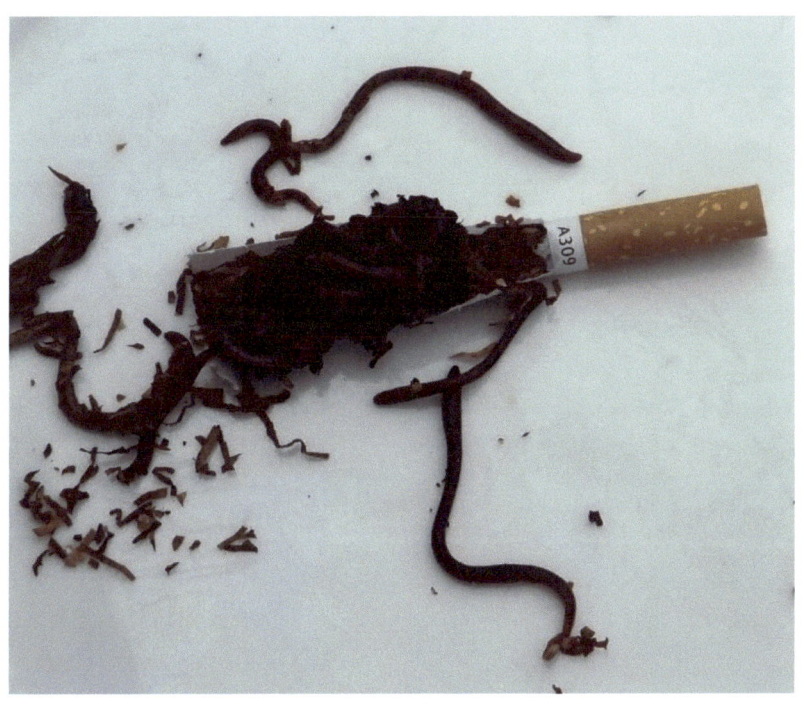

Cigarettes wormed their way into your life.

STOP now so cancer doesn't worm its way into you.

Yuck, YUCK!   Enjoy tasting healthy food again.

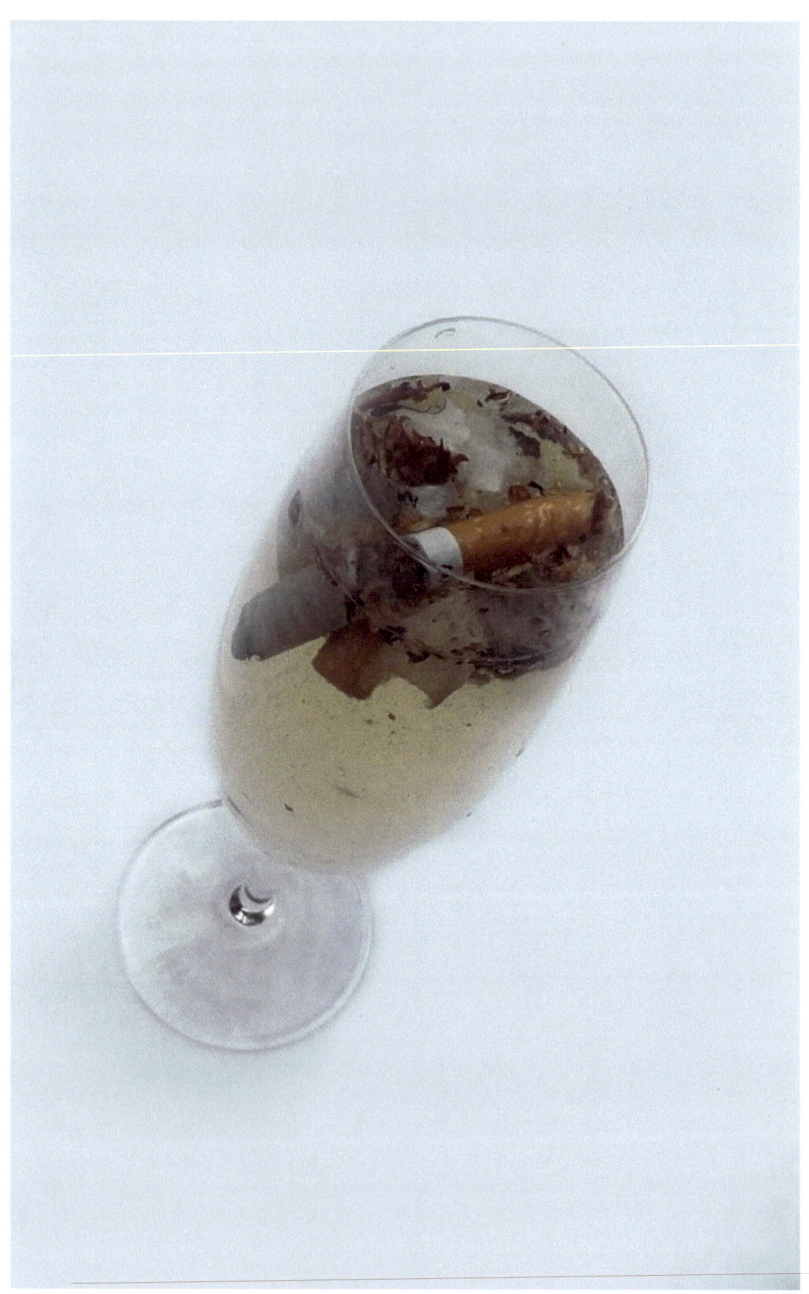

STOP treating yourself like a filter!

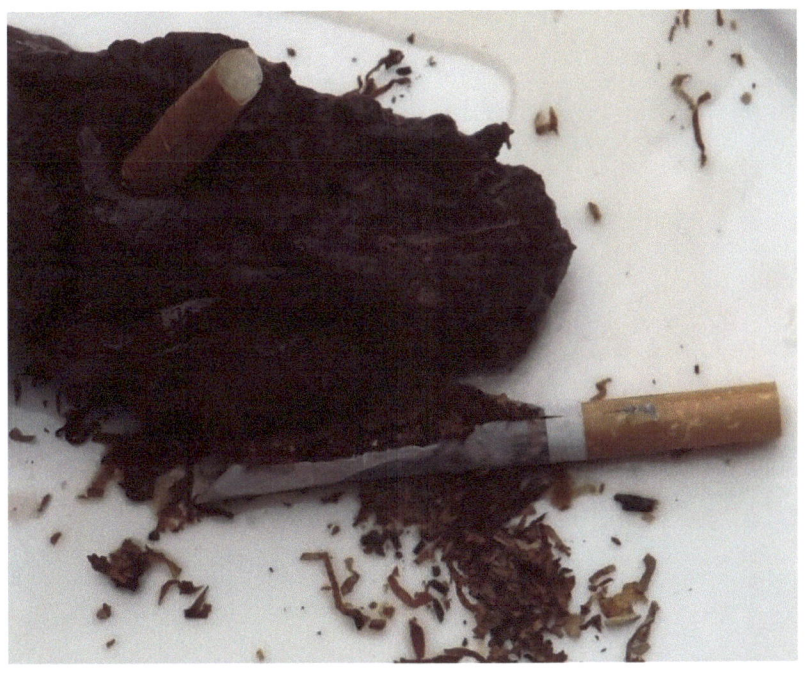

Cigarettes are SHIT !

Instructions:

Are you ready to stop smoking? If you really want to get rid of that old addiction you will need:

1. this book.

2. something that *smells* bad to YOU (e.g. rotten egg, rancid oil, off milk, diluted cleaning product, rotten garbage or compost, etc.).

3. (optional) something that *tastes* bad to YOU personally or e.g. smelly goats cheese, over-ripe bananas, Tabasco sauce, whatever turns you off.

PROCEDURE

First:
Look at the picture of the cigarettes on the first page. Note how much you would want one (on a scale from 1 to 10).

Second:
Put the food you hate in your mouth and smell the substance that revolts you while looking at all of the pictures in the book. Spend at least a minute on each of the pictures you find revolting. Read. Imagine a better life free of that old addiction.

Third:
Look at the first picture again and notice how little you need it now (on a scale of 1 to 10).

Fourth:
Keep the book with you when you go shopping to remind yourself that you no longer smoke. Don't buy any cigarettes.

Fifth:

Remember to **PAUSE:**

Punch the air 100 times or go for a walk etc. at times when you used to smoke. This is to pause and avoid those revolting toxin sticks. You can get a good feeling from exercise instead. Take time out for yourself.

Air can be breathed in deeply to relax you and fill you with energy and evaporate those old cravings. Imagine stress leaving you as you exhale.

Understand that it was the deep inhaling that relaxed you and that after three days there is no nicotine left in your system. Water can be drunk to wash away any future shadows of cravings.

Search for pressure points (like the one between your eyebrows) to relax and calm yourself.

Ensure that cigarettes are unavailable to you. Don't keep any. Throw them away (instead of your life).

Welcome to a new life where you have control over those old addictions you used to have. You can remember to live free of nicotine.

Disclaimer: no guarantees given for effectiveness. Pictures are planned to supplement the effect of an existing desire to stop smoking, and help you to help yourself reduce cravings for it and find better things to do instead. Use common sense when selecting substances that smell or taste bad to supplement the therapy. Ensure they are safe, non-toxic and non-allergenic. When in doubt consult your counsellor or doctor.

The End   =>   the first day of the rest of your life

www.ingramcontent.com/pod-product-compliance
Lightning Source LLC
Chambersburg PA
CBHW041618180526
45159CB00002BC/916